Mitochondria Health

Unlocking the Power within

Dr. Dave Wilson

Copyright © 2024 by Dr. Dave Wilson.
All rights reserved. No part of this publication may be reproduced, distributed, or transmitted in any form or by any means, without the prior written permission of the publisher.

Disclaimer: The information in this book is not meant to be used as medical advice; rather, it is meant only for educational reasons. It is not intended to replace expert medical supervision or be used for diagnosis. It is recommended that you address any medical condition with a healthcare provider before using any of the provided information. Both the publisher and the author release themselves from any liability regarding any injury allegedly resulting from anything included in this book.

Table of Contents:

KEY INSIGHT

Unleashing Inner Strength: An Exploration into Mitochondrial Health

Imagine an extensive web of minuscule power plants buzzing within each and every cell of your body, supplying energy to every thought, movement, and heartbeat. These are the amazing organelles called mitochondria, not some kind of legendary engine. They are sophisticated dance floors where life's essential functions pirouette—much more than basic batteries—and they hold the secret to our longevity, vitality, and overall health.

These minuscule wonders were pushed to the back of biology textbooks for many years. However, a new revolution has brought them to light and exposed their significant influence on our wellbeing. Researchers are currently deciphering the mitochondrial health mysteries, opening the door to a time when we will be able to utilize their potential to enhance our quality of life.

Understanding the underlying factors that shape our inner environment is the goal of this voyage into mitochondrial health. It concerns:

Uncovering the secrets of their composition and operation: Investigating the complex creases in their membranes, learning about the energy-producing electron transport chain, and studying how they interact with other cells.

Aware of their impact on several facets of health: Mitochondria are essential to our general health, controlling everything from metabolism and immunity to aging and brain function.

Uncovering the connection between disease and mitochondrial dysfunction: exposing how these powerhouses' defects can be linked to a variety of afflictions, from metabolic diseases like diabetes and obesity to neurodegenerative disorders like Parkinson's and Alzheimer's.

Unlocking the potential of mitochondrial medicine: Investigating state-of-the-art studies on gene editing, mitochondrial replacement therapy, and lifestyle modifications that could transform the medical field and provide us the ability to regain control over our health.

Mitochondrial health is a personal empowerment journey, not just a scientific endeavor. Understanding these internal essential engines allows us to reach new heights of resilience, vigor, and wellbeing. This is a call to action to set out on a journey of exploration, learn more about the fascinating world of mitochondria, and unleash your inner potential.

Ready to take up the revolution? Join us as we continue to explore the fascinating world of mitochondria, uncovering their secrets, revealing their function in both health and sickness, and uncovering the fascinating prospects that await in the field of mitochondrial medicine.

PHASE 1

Demystifying the Mitochondrial Marvels

Uncovering the Secrets of Mitochondrial Marvels: An Intense Overview of Cellular Superstars

Have you ever wondered what propels every thought, every heartbeat, and every muscle contraction? Deep within your cells, in small, active organelles known as mitochondria, is where the solution is found. These are complex dance floors where the tango of life unfolds, not just energy factories. But in the midst of the technical diagrams and scientific jargon, these cellular powerhouses are frequently left mysterious. Be at ease, inquisitive voyager! The purpose of this crash course is to explain the wonders of mitochondria.

Organization Revealed: Picture a teardrop with a smooth, shield-like outer membrane. A captivating landscape opens up inside. The cristae of the inner membrane, folded onto themselves like mountain ranges, enhance surface area for energy production. Tucked away in these creases is the electron transport chain, a molecular conveyor belt that converts our food into ATP, the energy source for our cells. Imagine it as a little electrical grid that is always humming to maintain the functionality of cells.

Extra Word of Wisdom: However, "powerhouse" is merely the beginning. As multifunctional organelles, mitochondria control calcium signaling for both nerve impulses and muscle contractions. They serve as the cell's cleaning crew, allowing damaged players to be removed by cell death.

Furthermore, they interact with the nucleus like expert negotiators, affecting gene expression and reshaping our basic biology.

Transformational Tango: Just as fascinating as the role mitochondria play is their story. These superpowers are old bacterial invaders, not inherent to our cells! They partnered symbiotically with our single-celled ancestors billions of years ago, providing them with a safe habitat in exchange for their energy expertise. Because of this evolutionary dance, sophisticated life emerged, and mitochondria are now essential to every heartbeat and thought that occurs in our minds.

Dual Role of DNA: The small genome, a circular strand of DNA separate from the nuclear DNA, is stored in each mitochondrion. Understanding the vulnerabilities of this mitochondrial DNA is essential, since mutations can result in a host of health issues. The mitochondrial code is being unraveled quickly by research, opening up new avenues for customized medicine and possible treatments.

From Course Books to Actualities: Our investigation into these wonders goes beyond dry technical terminology. We'll look at actual cases of diseases ranging from metabolic conditions like diabetes to neurological conditions like Parkinson's that are caused by mitochondrial malfunction. We'll also dispel the myths and false beliefs that have surrounded mitochondria for ages as we examine historical and cultural viewpoints on them.

Inspiring Decisions: It takes more than just theoretical understanding to demystify these powerhouses—it takes empowerment. We'll provide you with helpful advice on how to maintain the health of your mitochondria through food, exercise, and lifestyle decisions. We can learn to maximize these internal engines' performance and so foster vitality, resilience, and overall well-being throughout our lifetimes by getting to know them.

Ready to:

Discover the secrets of mitochondrial DNA and its function in health; Take in the breathtaking dance of the electron transport chain.

Examine the connection between a number of diseases and mitochondrial malfunction.

Learn useful techniques to support your inner superheroes.

This is only a small sampling of the fascinating realm of mitochondria. Follow along as we uncover their mysteries, one engrossing chapter at a time, in our quest for a stronger, healthier you!

Chapter 1: Introducing the Mighty Mitochondria

Presenting the Powerful Mitochondria: Enabling the Circular Motion of Life

Ever wondered about the silent engines that power every thought, action, and heartbeat inside every single cell in your body? These are not fantastical devices, but the amazing organelles called "mitochondria". They're sophisticated dance floors where the tango of life unfolds, far more than basic batteries, and they hold the secret to our vitality, health, and even longevity.

Consider looking into a world that is minuscule. Rather to being a lifeless wasteland, you find a thriving city driven by microscopic, dynamic power plants called mitochondria. They are the conductors of a cellular symphony, coordinating essential activities to keep you alive and well. These are not just energy manufacturers.

Organization Revealed: Every mitochondrion has the appearance of a smooth teardrop and is shielded by a smooth membrane. A captivating landscape opens up inside. The inner membrane's 'cristae' fold like mountain ranges to optimize surface area for 'energy production'. Tucked away in these creases is the 'electron transport chain', a molecular conveyor belt that converts our food into ATP, the energy source for our cells. Imagine it as a little electrical grid that is always humming to maintain the functionality of cells.

Outside of Batteries: However, mitochondria are much more than just metabolic engines. They control 'calcium signaling', which affects nerve impulses and muscle contractions. They serve as the cell's cleaning crew, allowing damaged players to be removed by cell death. Additionally, they interact with the nucleus like expert messengers, affecting gene expression and reshaping our very biology.

Legacy of Evolution: Just as fascinating as the role mitochondria play is their story. These superpowers are old bacterial invaders, not inherent to our cells! They partnered symbiotically with our single-celled ancestors billions of years ago, providing them with a safe habitat in exchange for their energy expertise. Because of this evolutionary dance, sophisticated life emerged, and mitochondria are now essential to every heartbeat and thought that occurs in our minds.

Myths Exposed: These enigmatic organelles have been the subject of myths throughout history. While some referred to them as "tiny furnaces," others simply saw them as energy manufacturers. However, the full intricacy of them and their enormous influence on human wellbeing are now being revealed by modern research.

The Adventure Commences: We've only just begun to delve into the fascinating realm of mitochondria. We'll explore their complex mechanisms in more detail, learn how they affect health and illness, and learn about the fascinating prospects for mitochondrial medicine in the following chapters.

Unveiling their structure, function, and vital role in cellular life.

Uncovering the Powerful Mitochondria: Composition, Role, and Life's Dance

There is a hidden world, a humming metropolis called 'mitochondria', located deep within each and every cell in your body. These are not just batteries; these are complex dance floors where life's tango plays out, coordinating a symphony of essential functions to keep you alive and well. Let us first examine the structure, function, and crucial role that these powerful mitochondria play in cellular life before delving into the intricacies.

A Modern Style: Picture a teardrop with a smooth, shield-like outer membrane. Inside, the scene opens up like a miniature wonderland. The cristae of the inner membrane, folded onto themselves like mountain ranges, enhance surface area for energy production. Tucked away in these creases is the electron transport chain, a molecular conveyor belt that converts our food into ATP, the energy source for our cells.

Imagine it as a little electrical grid that is always humming to maintain the functionality of cells.

Extra Word of Wisdom: However, "powerhouse" is merely the beginning. Within the cellular ballet, mitochondria have multiple roles. They control calcium signaling, which affects nerve impulses and muscle contractions. They serve as the cell's cleaning crew, allowing damaged players to be removed by cell death. Furthermore, they interact with the nucleus like expert negotiators, affecting gene expression and reshaping our basic biology.

Transformational Tango: Just as fascinating as the role mitochondria play is their story. These superpowers are old bacterial invaders, not inherent to our cells! They partnered symbiotically with our single-celled ancestors billions of years ago, providing them with a safe habitat in exchange for their energy expertise. Because of this evolutionary dance, sophisticated life emerged, and mitochondria are now essential to every heartbeat and thought that occurs in our minds.

Dual Role of DNA: The small genome, a circular strand of DNA separate from the nuclear DNA, is stored in each mitochondrion. Understanding the vulnerabilities of this mitochondrial DNA is essential, since mutations can result in a host of health issues. The mitochondrial code is being unraveled quickly by research, opening up new avenues for customized medicine and possible treatments.

The Effect of Ripples: There may be severe repercussions if these titans of industry fall. Numerous illnesses, including neurological conditions like Parkinson's and Alzheimer's as well as metabolic conditions like diabetes and obesity, have been related to mitochondrial malfunction. The secret to opening up fresh possibilities for prevention and treatment is comprehending how these faults happen.

Inspiring Decisions: Empowerment is the goal of demystifying these powerful engines, not just theoretical understanding. We'll provide you with helpful advice on how to maintain the health of your mitochondria through food, exercise, and lifestyle decisions. We can learn to maximize these internal engines' performance and so foster vitality, resilience, and overall well-being throughout our lifetimes by getting to know them.

Chapter 2: The Dance of Energy Production

The Energy Production Dance: A Microscopic Tango Performed by Your Cells

The most intriguing dance floor in your body is found within the very fabric of your cells; forget disco balls and flashing lights. Greetings from the little powerhouses known as the mitochondria, where the tango of energy production takes place, supplying energy to every movement, thought, and heartbeat.

The Cha Cha Electron: Picture a molecular conveyor belt winding its way through the creases in the membrane of the mitochondria. This is the maestro of the tango of energy production, the electron transport chain. Glucose and other fuel molecules enter effortlessly, prepared for breakdown. Little dancers with a lot of punch, electrons are taken out and accompanied hand in hand by a number of protein companions as they move up the chain.

Power Play and Proton Pumps: A type of energy dam is created as the electrons pump protons across the membrane with each step, resulting in an electrochemical gradient. Protons unleash their stored energy when they rush back through membrane channels, which fuels the synthesis of ATP, the cell's universal energy unit. It produces electricity to power the cellular city in a manner similar to water rushing through a turbine.

The Grand Finale of Oxygen: Without the last flourish, oxygen, this tango would not be complete. This essential gas stabilizes the process and stops the production of dangerous free radicals by acting as the electron acceptor at the end of the chain. The oxygen guarantees a constant supply of ATP for all the cellular operations that keep you running and make the dance flow smoothly.

Beyond the Fundamentals: However, there is more to the dance of energy creation than merely graceful moves. It's an exquisitely synchronized performance, with each protein partner contributing significantly. Genetic mutations or environmental factors can cause disruptions in the cycle that result in energy deficiencies, which can affect organ function and contribute to a variety of disorders.

Unleashing the Inner Powerhouse: Gaining an understanding of this dance's nuances enables us to support the health of our mitochondria. We may maximize the internal tango, fostering resilience and energy, by controlling stress, exercising, and selecting the correct fuel (consider meals high in nutrients!).

Your mitochondria's tango of energy production is proof of life's wonderful design. We may release the power within and dance our way to a better, more vibrant version of ourselves by recognizing its beauty and comprehending how it functions.

Exploring the electron transport chain and ATP generation, the fuel of life.

A Comprehensive Look at the Powerhouse: Investigating the Electron Transport Chain and the Production of ATP

After seeing the fascinating dance floor of the cristae and peeping through the shimmering membrane of the powerful mitochondria, it's time to focus in on the minute processes that power our own existence: the electron transport chain and the synthesis of ATP, the fuel of life.

The Sequence of Events: Imagine a race between molecules—a molecular relay—snaking along the inner membrane's folds. Our speedy runners, electrons, are champions with a baton who are taken out of food molecules like glucose. Together, they set out on an exciting adventure through a sequence of protein complexes that serve as checkpoints along the chain.

Increasing the Force: The proteins not only transmit the baton with each handoff, but they also plan an important side act. By forcing protons across the membrane, they create an electrochemical gradient, which functions as a type of cellular battery that can store potential energy. Imagine it as water pooling behind a dam, waiting to release its pressure.

The Grand Entrance of Oxygen: The last act now begins. The ultimate acceptor of electrons, oxygen, enters the stage. When electrons arrive at their destination, they mix with protons and oxygen to create water. But this is the big finish, not just a lovely bow! 'ATP' is produced as protons rush back through membrane channels, propelled by the gradient they assisted in creating. This process releases a surge of energy.

ATP: The Global Money: Adenosine triphosphate, or ATP, is the unit of account for energy inside cells. It functions like small fuel packets, powering everything from nerve impulses to protein synthesis to muscle contraction. The cellular city comes to a complete stop in the absence of ATP, underscoring the vital function of this little power source.

Beyond the Fundamentals: This complex dance is a strictly regulated performance, not merely a diagram from a textbook. Every protein complex has a distinct melody, and any deviation from this might result in energy deficiencies with far-reaching effects. Numerous diseases can be caused by genetic abnormalities, environmental conditions, or even lifestyle decisions that throw off the chain.

Giving the Dance Strength: However, knowing the electron transport chain is about empowerment rather than just doom and misery. Through a nutrient-dense diet, exercise, and stress management, we may optimize the dance within our mitochondria and guarantee a consistent supply of ATP for a vibrant and healthy existence.

Investigate the connection between diseases such as metabolic and neurodegenerative disorders and mitochondrial malfunction.

Learn about state-of-the-art studies on chain manipulation for possible therapeutic interventions. Discover doable tactics to ignite your inner superpowers and bring them to their greatest potential.

The production of ATP and the electron transport chain are graceful examples of the complexity and power of life at its most basic level. We may unleash their potential, move to the beat of life, and forge ahead on our path to a stronger, healthier future by recognizing their subtleties and vulnerabilities.

Chapter 3: Beyond Batteries: Mitochondria's Diverse Roles

Without Batteries: Exposing the Orchestra Inside: The Various Functions of Mitochondria

Put an end to bulky automobile batteries; your cells' powerhouses function more like expert conductors, coordinating a symphony of essential functions that go far beyond simple energy generation. As the electron transport chain produces the energy (ATP) needed to sustain our movement, thought, and breathing, mitochondria perform a variety of roles in the grand scheme of life.

Calcium Cacophony: Visualize microscopic cymbals that are regulated by mitochondria. These superpowers control calcium signaling, an essential nerve and muscle impulse conductor. Like drumbeats, they produce calcium ions, which cause muscle fibers to flex and send impulses that speed through neurons. Tremors, cardiac issues, and muscle weakness can all result from dysregulated calcium transmission.

The Cleaning Team: Because life isn't always pretty, mitochondria take care of the grubby stuff. They enable "cell death, which is an infected or damaged cell's natural process of self-destruction. They preserve tissue integrity and stop the spread of cellular disarray by eliminating these dysfunctional players. Autoimmune disorders and cancer may be exacerbated by impaired cell death.

Crying out to the Core: In any symphony, communication is essential, and mitochondria are expert communicators. Through signaling molecules, they exchange information with the nucleus, the cell's command center. This conversation affects gene expression, determining which genes are activated and inactive, and eventually determining how our body functions and reacts to external stimuli. This communication can be hampered by mitochondrial malfunction, which may have an effect on immunity, metabolism, and even aging.

Lover of Antioxidants: Free radicals cause havoc in cellular harmony, much like off-key notes in music. As experts in antioxidants, mitochondria use their enzymes like tools to counteract these dangerous substances. This shields cells against oxidative stress, which is a major cause of aging and a number of illnesses. Cells that have compromised antioxidant defenses are more susceptible to harm and malfunction.

Survival Encore: This varied repertory bears witness to the intriguing history of mitochondria. These superpowers aren't indigenous to our cells; billions of years ago, ancient bacteria invaded our cells and developed a symbiotic relationship. Because of this evolutionary encore, complex life emerged, and mitochondria are now essential to human survival.

Unlocking the Potential: Knowing the complete extent of their responsibilities enables us to develop these adaptable performers. We can support their many functions and promote resilience and general health by eating foods high in antioxidants, practicing stress management, and getting regular exercise.

Examine the intricacies of gene expression regulation by mitochondria, calcium signaling, and pathways leading to cell death.

Discover the connection between diseases other than those that are typically associated with energy.

Learn about state-of-the-art studies on utilizing mitochondria's varied capabilities for therapeutic interventions. Discover doable tactics to synchronize your cellular symphony for optimal health and unleash your inner orchestra.

Mitochondria are much more than just biological batteries; they are combined messengers, conductors, and sanitization teams. Through recognizing their adaptability and comprehending their influence on our health, we can unleash their potential and arrange a lively, wholesome tune in the magnificent spectacle of life.

Delving into their influence on metabolism, calcium signaling, cell death, and aging.

Dive Further: How the Symphony of Life Is Orchestrated by Mitochondria

We have shown the fascinating dance of energy production that occurs inside mitochondria, as well as their function as cellular conductors and wide range of uses beyond being just batteries. Let's now take a closer look at the complex ways these superpowers affect important functions, including metabolism, calcium signaling, cell death, and even aging.

Masters of Metabolism: Consider mitochondria as small factories that produce ATP, the cellular currency, by breaking down the fuels we eat, such as glucose and lipids. This metabolic dance is a meticulously choreographed performance that involves more than just raw force. Mitochondria optimize fuel consumption by adjusting energy output according to cellular requirements. Changes in this metabolic dance can cause a variety of issues, ranging from diabetes and obesity to neurological illnesses.

Calcium Cacophony: Recall the cymbals that mitochondria control? Their complex concerto is calcium signaling. These metabolic powerhouses control nerve impulses, enzyme activity, and even muscle contractions by releasing and reabsorbing calcium ions. An imbalance in the cellular score might result from dysregulated calcium signaling, which can cause tremors, muscular weakness, and potentially cardiac arrhythmias. Novel treatments for neurological and cardiovascular disorders may be made possible by gaining a better understanding of how mitochondria regulate calcium.

The Technique of Giving Up: Although it's sometimes viewed as a tragic conclusion, cell death plays a vital role in cellular play. This process of apoptosis—programmed self-destruction—is mostly mediated by mitochondria. By triggering the breakdown of cellular machinery by enzymes, they guarantee the elimination of harmed or infected players. The hallmark of cancer is unchecked cell growth, which can be caused by impaired apoptosis. On the other hand, excessive cell death can cause tissue degradation and autoimmune disorders. We may be able to find novel approaches to tissue regeneration and cancer treatment by comprehending the role of mitochondria in apoptosis.

The Internal Clock: The ultimate conclusion of life's symphony, aging, is impacted by our inner superpowers as well. As mitochondrial dysfunction worsens over time, oxidative stress rises, and energy production is hindered. This ultimately leads to the aging process by promoting tissue malfunction and cellular deterioration. However, studies are revealing ways to adjust antioxidant defenses and mitochondrial activity, which may provide methods for delaying the aging process and encouraging healthy aging.

Empowering Performance: Being aware of mitochondria's many effects enables us to take charge of our own well-being. Through dietary choices that are high in nutrients, stress management techniques, and consistent exercise, we can enhance their metabolic efficiency, control calcium signaling, enhance cell death processes, and possibly slow down the aging process.

Learn more about the precise processes governing mitochondrial control in cell death, metabolism, calcium signaling, and aging. Investigate state-of-the-art studies focusing on these pathways for therapeutic interventions in a range of illnesses.

Acquire useful tactics to enhance mitochondrial performance and foster adaptability throughout these crucial procedures. Discover the secrets of long life and investigate how mitochondria may help to encourage aging in a healthy way.

We can better understand mitochondria's strength and complexity by exploring the myriad ways they affect life's fundamental functions. With this understanding, we may actively participate in the magnificent symphony of life, guaranteeing a harmonious performance inside our cells and fostering vigorous health all the way through our trip.

Chapter 4: A Symphony of Communication

The vital organelles, known as mitochondria, are involved in both energy production and cellular metabolism. The procedures by which mitochondria transmit information and bioenergetic potential to nearby mitochondria and other organelles are referred to as mitochondrial communication. In order to preserve mitochondrial quality control and guarantee normal cellular activity, this communication is essential. Numerous stressors, such as physical inactivity, infections, dietary changes, or mental strain, might impair mitochondrial communication. Mitokines, also known as myomitokines, are substances that mitochondria in the heart and skeletal muscles utilize to communicate with other cells or organs. Numerous illnesses, such as cancer and neurodegeneration, are directly linked to mitochondrial stress and aging. It is possible that mitokines facilitate intercellular mitochondrial communication, but more research is needed to confirm this.

Understanding how mitochondria interact with the nucleus and other organelles.

Beyond Solo Performances: The Intersection of the Nucleus and Organelle Orchestra with the Mitochondrial Network

We have looked at the fascinating dance of energy production that occurs within mitochondria, their wide range of functions that extend beyond batteries, and their significant impact on important cellular functions. However, these powerhouses don't operate in a vacuum; rather, they're a part of a vibrant cellular metropolis that interacts and works along with the nucleus, which serves as the city's command center, and other organelles. Let's explore this complex network and learn how mitochondria communicate and operate together with other cells.

Dialogue from Core to Powerhouse: Envision a direct phone line connecting the power plant (mitochondria) and the CEO's office (nucleus).

'Signaling molecules' help to facilitate this essential channel of communication. These messengers carry instructions from the nucleus, which controls mitochondrial activity according to cellular requirements. For instance, the nucleus can send signals to the mitochondria to increase ATP production if energy demands increase. This complex conversation guarantees effective resource distribution and stable cellular operation.

Masters of the Mitochondrion: However, the exchange of ideas is two-way. In addition, mitochondria communicate with the nucleus about the state of the cell and the amount of energy they are producing. The nucleus can modify gene expression through this feedback loop, which affects the synthesis of proteins required for mitochondrial function. For instance, the nucleus may produce more repair enzymes if it detects damage to the mitochondria. In order to respond to external stresses and preserve cellular homeostasis, this two-way communication is essential.

Symphonic Orchestra: Mitochondria converse with other organelles in addition to the nucleus. They trade endoplasmic reticulum and peroxisomes for metabolites, the tiny chemicals that power cellular functions. They work together in the transport of proteins and lipids with the Golgi apparatus. Furthermore, they influence the shape and motility of cells by interacting with the cytoskeleton. Smooth cellular operations and effective resource use are guaranteed by this complex web of relationships.

Beyond Harmony: Implications of Disturbance: The ramifications of a breakdown in cellular network connectivity might be extensive. Abruptions in the communication between the nucleus and mitochondria can result in energy deficiencies, which can affect organ performance and be a factor in a number of disorders. Analogously, compromised connections with additional organelles have the potential to impede essential metabolic routes and cellular functions. Comprehending their interdependence is essential to formulating efficacious treatment approaches for intricate illnesses.

Empowering the Network: Our understanding of how mitochondria cooperate and communicate gives us the ability to facilitate their interactions. We can enhance the performance of the organelle symphony and encourage healthy cellular communication by exercising regularly, eating nutrient-rich foods, and controlling stress. This all-encompassing strategy can support general health and fortify against illnesses stemming from discord in the cells.

Understanding the interdependence of our cells helps us to better appreciate the crucial role mitochondria play in preserving health and wellbeing. By using this perspective, we can cultivate harmony within our cellular network and unlock the potential to grow, thereby taking an active role in the grand performance of life.

The Shadow Side: When Powerhouses Falter

The vital organelles, known as mitochondria, are involved in both energy production and cellular metabolism. Numerous illnesses, such as cancer, noncommunicable chronic diseases, and dementia, can be brought on by mitochondrial malfunction. The procedures by which mitochondria transmit information and bioenergetic potential to nearby mitochondria and other organelles are referred to as mitochondrial communication. In order to preserve mitochondrial quality control and guarantee normal cellular activity, this communication is essential. Mitokines, also known as myomitokines, are substances that mitochondria in the heart and skeletal muscles utilize to communicate with other cells or organs. Mitochondrial stress is intimately linked to aging and can be caused by a number of stressors, such as infections, physical inactivity, changes in diet, or mental strain. It is possible that mitokines facilitate intercellular mitochondrial communication, but more research is needed to confirm this. Avoiding stressors and supplying the required substrates, such as vitamins, minerals, and antioxidants, to sustain mitochondrial function are crucial for maintaining healthy mitochondria.

Chapter 5: Mitochondrial Dysfunction: A Cascade of Consequences

Mitochondrial Mayhem: The Fall of the Superpowers

Imagine a thriving metropolis fueled by an impressive central generator. Everything is buzzing with activity because energy is always flowing. However, what occurs if the generator falters and sputters? Pandemonium spreads, affecting every area of the city. This is essentially the tale of mitochondrial dysfunction, a disorder in which the engines of our cells malfunction, resulting in a series of events that can have a significant negative influence on our health.

Power Overshadowed: An 'energy crisis' is the most common direct result of mitochondrial malfunction. The complex dance of the electron transport chain falters, resulting in a reduction in the synthesis of ATP, the energy currency of cells. This lack of energy causes organs and tissues to hunger, which affects basic cellular functions as well as brain and muscular activities. Imagine buildings becoming dark and traffic lights flickering; such is the cellular environment under the influence of mitochondrial malfunction.

Debilitating Attack: Dangerous free radicals, which are reactive molecules similar to cellular vandals, start to amass when the electron transport chain breaks down. When the antioxidant defenses are overpowered by this oxidative stress, proteins, DNA, and delicate cellular machinery are damaged. It resembles a metropolis destroyed by uncontrollably spreading flames, with essential infrastructure collapsing beneath the damage.

Calcium Soundscape: Recall the complex calcium signaling that mitochondria arranged? The delicate balance is upset when these formidable figures falter. Muscle contractions, neuronal impulses, and even enzyme activity are disrupted when calcium ions seep out of the chambers that are meant for them. Cellular functions become chaotic as a result of this calcium din, much like a city's communication system breaking down due to an overload of static.

Demolition Derby for Cells: Mitochondria are essential for the elimination of damaged players during programmed cell death in healthy cells. However, in cases of dysfunction, this process may become chaotic. Apoptosis, or controlled self-destruction, may be compromised, which could allow injured cells to survive and possibly contribute to unchecked cell growth, which is a defining feature of cancer. On the other hand, excessive cell death can happen and impair organs and tissues, similar to structures collapsing before their time.

Disease Chain Reaction: Wide-ranging disorders are linked to mitochondrial malfunction, which has far-reaching effects. The malfunctioning of our cellular powerhouses has been connected to a number of maladies, including metabolic diseases like diabetes and obesity, cardiovascular diseases, neurodegenerative disorders like Parkinson's and Alzheimer's, and even chronic fatigue syndrome. Similar to a domino effect, a first energy deficiency sets off a series of disturbances that affect different organ systems.

Hope Is Shining: There is more to the story of mitochondrial malfunction than just death and despair. The field of research is moving quickly forward, revealing the complex workings of these superpowers and investigating possible treatments. Scientists are working nonstop to maximize communication channels, target antioxidant defenses, and use gene therapy to fully use mitochondria for the benefit of human health.

Building Up Our Inner Superstars: We can choose our lifestyles to empower our inner powerhouses while research is ongoing. We can promote mitochondrial health and resilience by eating a diet high in nutrients, controlling our stress levels, and exercising frequently. It's analogous to giving the city's generator the proper fuel, consistent upkeep, and a secure operating environment.

Knowing the effects of mitochondrial dysfunction gives us the power to speak out for ourselves and take an active role in our healthcare process. We can unleash the potential for a healthier, more vibrant future by collaborating with healthcare professionals and supporting ongoing research to negotiate the complexity of these cellular powerhouses.

Investigating the link between mitochondrial defects and various diseases.

The Shadowy Labyrinth: Exposing the Connection Between Disease and Mitochondrial Defects

The powerful mitochondria thump and dance deep within our cells, supplying energy for each and every heartbeat, thought, and movement. However, what occurs when these titans falter? The effects can be extensive, creating a complex network of links to different illnesses. In this exploration, we'll explore the complex world of mitochondrial defects and how they may be related to a variety of illnesses.

From Blackouts to Internal Disorders: Imagine the unexpected darkness that descends upon a bustling metropolis. This is similar to the energy crisis that arises in cells when abnormalities in the mitochondria cause disruptions in the electron transport chain, which is the complex dance responsible for producing ATP, the cellular energy currency. This energy deficiency doesn't stay in one place; rather, it spreads, affecting the functions of important organs and setting off a series of unfavorable consequences.

Oxidative Onslaught: As the electrical grid collapses, dangerous free radicals that resemble cellular vandals start to build up. The antioxidant defenses are overpowered by this oxidative stress, which wreaks havoc on fragile proteins, DNA, and cellular components. It resembles a metropolis destroyed by uncontrolled fires, with essential infrastructure falling apart.

Calcium Soundscape: Recall the complex calcium signaling that mitochondria arranged? The delicate balance is upset when these formidable figures falter. When calcium ions escape from the spaces allotted to them, enzyme function, neuronal signals, and muscle contractions are interfered with. Cellular functions become chaotic as a result of this calcium cacophony, much like a city's communication system failing under a deluge of static.

Disease Chain Reaction: Let's now investigate the complex relationships that exist between these cellular disturbances and particular diseases:

Diseases of the Nervous System: Because our brains require so much energy, they are especially susceptible to mitochondrial malfunction. Mutations in mitochondrial DNA have been connected to disorders such as Parkinson's and Alzheimer's, which can result in reduced energy generation and oxidative stress, which can ultimately lead to neuronal death.

Metabolic Disorders: Defects in the mitochondria can also be seen in diabetes and obesity. Dysfunctional mitochondria that struggle to turn food into energy are the cause of impaired glucose metabolism and insulin signaling, which are frequently linked to these disorders.

Diseases of the Heart: Regular ATP production is essential for heart function. Mitochondrial abnormalities have the potential to cause arrhythmias, heart failure, weakening of the heart muscle, and disruption of electrical signaling.

Condition of Chronic Fatigue: The crippling exhaustion that characterizes this illness may be related to deficiencies in mitochondrial energy, which leave sufferers exhausted and unable to carry out daily tasks.

Deconstructing the Mysteries: The intricate network of relationships between mitochondrial abnormalities and disease is being actively unraveled by research. Mutations in mitochondrial DNA are being identified by genetic investigations, cellular dysfunction is being shown by sophisticated imaging tools, and novel medicines are being investigated to target particular pathways and maybe lessen the effects.

Building Up Our Inner Superstars: While scientific research is ongoing, we may strengthen our inner superpowers by making certain lifestyle decisions. Stress reduction, a nutrient-rich diet, and regular exercise can all support the best possible mitochondrial resilience and health. It's analogous to giving the city's generator the proper fuel, consistent upkeep, and a secure operating environment.

We can learn a lot about the relationship between mitochondrial abnormalities and different diseases, which helps us make better decisions about our own health and wellbeing. This information gives us the ability to speak up for ourselves, actively engage in healthcare decisions, and enthusiastically welcome new research. Recall that the dark web of mitochondrial malfunction is beginning to clear, opening the door to a day when we can utilize these cellular engines to achieve better health and a more energetic existence.

Chapter 6: Neurodegenerative Diseases: A Mitochondrial Connection

The Dimming Symphony: Investigating the Role of Mitochondria in Neurodegenerative Illnesses

The electrical symphony of the human brain is a vivid tapestry of interconnected neurons. However, if this symphony breaks down, the effects can be disastrous. Alzheimer's, Parkinson's, and ALS are examples of neurodegenerative diseases that throw a long shadow, making it harder to remember things, move around, and eventually, live. Mitochondria, the powerful powerhouses found within our cells, have emerged as a vital role, even if the origins of these complicated illnesses are yet unknown.

Crisis in Energy at the Command Center: Consider a sudden power outage that affects the brain, the organ in our body that uses the most energy. This is precisely what occurs in neurodegenerative diseases: a "deficit in ATP, the cellular energy currency, results from mitochondrial malfunction that upsets the delicate dance of the electron transport chain. Fuel-starved neurons start to malfunction, communication networks break down, and the rhythm of cognitive activity begins to wane.

Oxidative Onslaught: As energy output falters, a hazardous byproduct known as 'free radicals' builds up. These cellular vandals damage sensitive proteins and DNA, hastening aging and playing a role in neuronal death. It resembles a city destroyed by uncontrolled fires, with the oxidative assault destroying the structural foundation of the brain.

Calcium Soundscape: Recall the complex calcium signaling that mitochondria arranged? This fine balance is upset when these titans falter. Leaking calcium ions from their assigned chambers can cause excitotoxicity, which can further damage or kill neurons as well as interfere with important nerve signals. The brain's communication network becomes chaotic due to this calcium cacophony, which muffles the once-vibrant symphony of movement and thought.

Membrane Landscapes and Disease Signatures: While the signs and symptoms of many neurodegenerative illnesses vary, mitochondrial dysfunction is frequently identified.

Alzheimer's Disease: The disorder is characterized by plaques and tangles that clog the brain. According to recent studies, oxidative stress and decreased mitochondrial protein function may be connected to these.

Disease Parkinson: The distinctive tremors and rigidity of Parkinson's are connected to the loss of dopamine-producing neurons in the brain. This mechanism has been linked to energy deficiencies and mitochondrial mutations.

Amyotrophic Lateral Sclerosis, or ALS: Motor neurons are impacted by this progressive neurodegenerative illness, which causes paralysis and muscle weakening. The role of mitochondrial dysfunction, especially disrupted calcium signaling, is becoming more widely acknowledged.

Solidarity in the Symphony: Even though research on neurodegenerative illnesses is still ongoing, knowledge of the mitochondrial relationship provides some optimism. Potential therapeutic approaches are being investigated in research.

Gene therapy: Targeting mutations in mitochondrial DNA may be able to prevent or slow down the progression of disease.

Antioxidants: Scavenging free radicals and reducing oxidative stress may protect neurons from mitochondrial damage.

Transplantation of mitochondria: This innovative approach offers a potential future treatment plan by substituting healthy mitochondria for malfunctioning ones.

Beyond the Microscope and Bench: Making lifestyle decisions that can empower our inner powerhouses might also be very important.

Nutrient-rich diet: Maintaining mitochondrial health can be achieved by giving the brain the proper fuel—a balanced diet high in antioxidants and vital nutrients.

Daily exercise: Physical activity increases the production of substances that protect against oxidative stress and enhances mitochondrial function. Stress management: Mitochondrial health may be adversely affected by prolonged stress. The general health of the brain can be enhanced by learning effective stress management techniques.

We give ourselves hope and knowledge by knowing the connection between mitochondria and neurodegenerative disorders. The brain's symphony may encounter difficulties, but by bolstering our cellular powerhouses and embracing continued study, we may be able to muffle these awful conditions and clear the path for a time when everyone can still enjoy the melodies of movement and memory.

Exploring the role of mitochondria in Parkinson's, Alzheimer's, and other brain disorders

The Mysterious Maze: Exposing the Mitochondrial Connection in Brain Illnesses

The mitochondria are small powerhouses that are tucked away among the busy avenues of neurons and synapses deep within the busy city of the brain. These biological motors hum and dance, powering every action, every thought, and every memory flicker. However, when these titans of industry stumble, the fallout can be catastrophic, leaving a lasting legacy of crippling brain diseases such as Parkinson's, Alzheimer's, and more.

Crisis in Energy at the Command Center: Imagine a busy city abruptly falling into darkness. This energy shortage is similar to what occurs in many brain illnesses, where the cellular currency of energy, "dearth of ATP, results from mitochondrial malfunction that impairs the electron transport chain. Lack of fuel causes neurons to stumble, disrupting communication networks and causing the lively symphony of cognition to lose rhythm. This energy crisis is a recurring theme in the mosaic of different brain illnesses.

Oxidative Onslaught: When the electrical grid malfunctions, 'free radicals'—a harmful byproduct—build up. These cellular vandals damage sensitive proteins and DNA, hastening aging and playing a role in neuronal death. It resembles a city destroyed by uncontrolled fires, with the oxidative assault destroying the structural foundation of the brain. This oxidative stress contributes significantly to the neurodegeneration seen in diseases such as Parkinson's and Alzheimer's.

Calcium Soundscape: Recall the complex calcium signaling that mitochondria arranged? This fine balance is upset when these titans falter. Leaking calcium ions from their assigned chambers can cause excitotoxicity, which can further damage or kill neurons as well as interfere with important nerve signals. The brain's communication network becomes chaotic due to this calcium cacophony, which muffles the once-vibrant symphony of movement and memory. The development of Parkinson's disease is specifically linked to this phenomenon.

Membrane Landscapes and Disease Signatures: Despite having different manifestations, mitochondrial dysfunction is frequently found in the following brain disorders:

Disease of Alzheimer: The distinctive brain tangles and plaques may be associated with oxidative stress and compromised mitochondrial protein function, which could impede the removal of these dangerous aggregates.

Disease Parkinson: The substantia nigra's dopamine-producing neurons have died, which is connected to the tremors and stiffness. This mechanism has been linked to energy deficiencies and mutations in mitochondrial DNA.

ALS: Amyotrophic Lateral Sclerosis Motor neurons are impacted by this progressive neurodegenerative illness, which causes paralysis and muscle weakening. The role of mitochondrial dysfunction, especially disrupted calcium signaling, is becoming more widely acknowledged.

Amid a Shadowy Labyrinth: A Glimmer of Hope: While research into the mitochondrial connection provides a glimmer of optimism, the fight against these debilitating brain illnesses is far from over. Potential therapeutic approaches are being thoroughly investigated by research.

Gene therapy: Targeting mutations in mitochondrial DNA may be able to prevent or slow down the progression of disease.

Antioxidants: Scavenging free radicals and reducing oxidative stress may protect neurons from mitochondrial damage.

Transplantation of mitochondria: This innovative approach offers a potential future treatment plan by substituting healthy mitochondria for malfunctioning ones.

Building Up Your Inner Powerhouses: Through lifestyle decisions, we can unleash our inner powerhouses outside of the bench and microscope.

Nutrient-rich diet: Maintaining mitochondrial health can be achieved by giving the brain the proper fuel—a balanced diet high in antioxidants and vital nutrients.

Daily exercise: Physical activity increases the production of substances that protect against oxidative stress and enhances mitochondrial function. Stress management: Mitochondrial health may be adversely affected by prolonged stress. The general health of the brain can be enhanced by learning effective stress management techniques.

Understanding the complex relationship between mitochondria and brain illnesses gives us hope and information. The vibrant city of the brain may face obstacles, but we can potentially turn down the volume on these debilitating conditions and pave the way for a future where everyone can continue to enjoy the lively symphony of cognitive function by embracing ongoing research, supporting our cellular powerhouses, and implementing preventive measures.

Chapter 7: Metabolic Mayhem: Mitochondria and Chronic Diseases

Metabolic Mayhem: Unveiling the Mitochondrial Link in Chronic Diseases: When the Inner Engines Sputter

Forget about renegade robots or extraterrestrial incursions; the greatest danger to our internal peace may be hiding inside each of our cells as microscopic power plants known as mitochondria. These metabolism-related engines can have far-reaching effects when they malfunction, causing a series of disturbances that show up as a variety of chronic illnesses. Fasten your seatbelts and join us as we explore the intriguing, if occasionally terrifying, realm of metabolic mayhem.

Power Overshadowed: Imagine a busy metropolis that is suddenly completely dark. This is similar to the internal energy crisis that arises in cells when a deficit in ATP, the cellular energy currency, results from mitochondrial malfunction interfering with the complex dance of the electron transport chain. This is not merely a localized blackout; it is a widespread phenomenon that affects organ function, sets off metabolic mayhem, and depletes tissues of oxygen.

Oxidative Onslaught: When energy production falters, dangerous 'free radicals' build up and cause havoc in the same way that cellular vandals do. The antioxidant defenses are overpowered by this oxidative stress, which damages DNA, proteins, and fragile cellular components. It resembles an uncontrollable wildfire destroying a city, with essential infrastructure collapsing beneath the poisonous damage.

Incorrect Metabolisms: Recall the complex metabolic processes that mitochondria manage. These systems go haywire when these powerhouses falter. When glucose metabolism is disrupted, cells find it difficult to use sugar as fuel, a condition known as "diabetes."An improper metabolism of fat leads to obesity and fatty liver disease. Additionally, sensitive hormone balances are upset, which may result in thyroid disorders and problems with reproduction.

Firestorm of Inflammation: The chaos of metabolism doesn't end there. Chronic low-grade inflammation is caused by mitochondrial malfunction and is akin to a cellular fire that spreads throughout the body. Numerous ailments, including autoimmune diseases like lupus and arthritis and neurodegenerative disorders like Parkinson's and Alzheimer's, are linked to this inflammatory firestorm.

Disease Chain Reaction: Let's now investigate the complex relationships that exist between this cellular turmoil and particular chronic illnesses:

Diabetes: Insulin resistance and poor glucose utilization are features of this common metabolic disease that are attributed to mitochondrial dysfunction.

Obesity: Impaired mitochondria make it difficult for fat to be burned off, which causes fat to accumulate and contributes to weight gain.

Autoimmune Diseases: Chronic inflammation brought on by mitochondrial dysfunction can attack healthy tissues, resulting in a variety of autoimmune conditions.

Cardiovascular Diseases: Impaired energy production within heart muscle cells weakens their function and increases the risk of heart failure and arrhythmias.

Hope Is Shining: There is more to the tale of metabolic mayhem than just dread and despair. The intricate network of links between mitochondrial malfunction and chronic illnesses is being actively unraveled by research with the aim of investigating possible therapeutic interventions.

Modulating metabolic pathways: New drugs and dietary approaches are being developed to optimize glucose and fat metabolism, addressing imbalances at their source.

Targeting oxidative stress: Antioxidant the rapies and lifestyle modifications can mitigate free radical damage and protect cellular infrastructure.

Supporting mitochondrial health: Stress reduction, nutrient-rich meals, and exercise can all help promote resilience and good mitochondrial function.

Finding Our Inner Power: While study is ongoing, we can use our lifestyle choices to unleash our inner powerhouses:

A diet rich in nutrients: By giving mitochondria the correct fuel—with a focus on antioxidants, nutritious foods, and healthy fats—we can support and nourish their function.

Daily exercise: Movement enhances energy production and mitochondrial biogenesis, which powers our inner engines more effectively.

Managing stress: Mitochondrial health may be adversely affected by prolonged stress. Discovering constructive coping mechanisms for stress can improve cellular health in general.

Gaining knowledge about the connection between chronic diseases and mitochondrial dysfunction allows us to make important decisions about our own health and wellbeing. This information gives us the ability to speak up for ourselves, actively engage in healthcare decisions, and enthusiastically welcome new research. Recall that the fight against metabolic mayhem is becoming more favorable. Through the encouragement of our inner engines and the adoption of a holistic approach, we may unleash our potential and create the foundation for a more vibrant, healthier future.

Unveiling how mitochondrial dysfunction contributes to diabetes, obesity, and related conditions.

Uncovering the Potential Within: How Diabetes, Obesity, and Other Conditions Are Caused by Mitochondrial Dysfunction

Hidden among the complex machinery of life, deep within our cells, are little power plants called mitochondria. These amazing organelles are in charge of producing energy, which is what powers our bodies. But when these tiny engines sputter and stall, it can lead to a plethora of chronic illnesses, including diabetes and obesity, among other health issues.

This is the tale of mitochondrial dysfunction, an obscure cause that lies beneath some of the modern world's most common health issues. It tells the story of unrealized potential, energy imbalances, and the incredible quest to release each cell's potential.

<u>The Life's Spark</u>:

There's more to mitochondria than just energy production. They affect cell signaling, control metabolism, and even contribute to apoptosis, or programmed cell death, and aging. Because they have their own DNA, which is a holdover from their time as free-living bacteria during their evolution, they are susceptible to damage and mutations.

<u>At Engine Sputtering Points</u>:

A number of factors, such as oxidative stress, genetic mutations, and environmental pollutants, can lead to mitochondrial malfunction. The fallout from these little powerhouses can have far-reaching effects.

Energy Shortage: The cellular currency of energy, ATP, is starved out of cells. Fatigue, and trouble controlling blood sugar can result from this.

Insulin Resistance: Insulin signaling is disrupted by impaired mitochondrial activity, which impairs glucose absorption and leads to type 2 diabetes.

Oxidative Stress: A build-up of free radicals resulting from mitochondrial failure can harm cells and tissues and exacerbate inflammation, a feature common to many chronic illnesses.

Obesity: Excessive fat intake can exacerbate malfunctioning mitochondria, affect energy production, and encourage weight gain. This can lead to a vicious cycle.

From Illness to Recovery:

The good news is that there is still hope for the tale of mitochondrial malfunction. By revealing the mysteries of these little powerhouses, we are opening the door to possible therapeutic interventions:

Dietary Interventions: Certain nutrients like L-carnitine and Coenzyme Q10 can support antioxidant defenses and mitochondrial energy production.

Lifestyle Modifications: Exercise, a nutritious diet high in antioxidants, and stress management can support mitochondrial health and function.

Emerging Therapies: To tackle the root cause of mitochondrial malfunction, research is looking into targeted drugs, gene therapy, and stem cell therapy.

Opening the Inner Power:

Being aware of mitochondrial dysfunction gives us the ability to control our health. By putting mitochondrial well-being first in our lifestyle decisions and investigating possible treatments, we can unleash the potential of every cell and provide the foundation for a more vibrant, healthy future.

The narrative is only getting started. We are in a position to fully realize the promise of mitochondria as research into this fascinating organ grows, not only to treat illness but also to enhance overall health and wellbeing. Our cells have power waiting to be unleashed; the secret

is to recognize and take care of the little engines
that ignite the spark of life.

Chapter 8: The Silent Culprit: Uncovering Genetic and Environmental Triggers

The Uncovering of Genetic and Environmental Triggers in Mitochondrial Health: The Silent Culprit

They quietly hum inside our cells, supplying energy for each heartbeat and every thought. However, when these little power plants, our mitochondria, malfunction, a host of health problems may appear out of the blue, leaving us to scrounge for solutions in the dark. This is the tale of mitochondrial dysfunction, an obscure cause that frequently lies at the heart of long-term illnesses including diabetes, obesity, and neurological disorders. Today, we go into the "quiet triggers, the genetic and environmental variables that upset these essential organelles' delicate balance, and the continuous pursuit of realizing their full potential.

The Fingerprint of DNA:

The condition of our mitochondria is largely influenced by our genetic composition. Mutations affecting mitochondrial DNA (mtDNA) can result in decreased energy generation and a heightened vulnerability to malfunction. These mutations can be inherited or acquired over time. Kearns-Sayre disease and Leber's hereditary optic neuropathy are two severe instances of how genetic errors can severely impair mitochondrial function.

Not Just in the Genes:

The environment is the paintbrush that shapes how the genetic blueprint is expressed, even though genetics has the blueprint. Mitochondrial dysfunction can be brought on by environmental causes such as exposure to pollutants, air pollution, and even some drugs. These variables frequently cause oxidative stress, which is the harmful accumulation of free radicals that overwhelms the mitochondria's natural defenses and sets off a downward spiral.

A Network of Relators:

Genetics and environment interact in a complicated tango. Particular genetic mutations have the potential to increase an individual's susceptibility to environmental stimuli, while specific environmental stressors have the potential to aggravate pre-existing mtDNA deficiencies. This complex network of factors emphasizes the necessity of a comprehensive strategy for comprehending and treating mitochondrial dysfunction.

Exposing the Offenders:

There is more work to be done to identify the quiet triggers. Advanced genetic sequencing techniques are being used in cutting-edge research to find new mtDNA mutations and discover environmental factors that cause mitochondrial decline. This increased comprehension opens the door to the creation of focused treatments and prophylactic measures.

Opening the Inner Power:

Although mitochondrial dysfunction is a major problem, there is also great hope for new treatment developments. Researchers are investigating ways to restore mitochondrial function and unleash the power within our cells by figuring out the genetic and environmental triggers. These methods include gene therapy, mitochondrial replacement approaches, and antioxidant-based therapies.

The Quiet Murderer Is No More:

Although mitochondrial dysfunction has remained hidden for far too long, its time is running out. We can stop, control, and possibly even reverse the harm by identifying the genetic and environmental causes. This goes beyond simply curing illnesses; it also involves bringing each cell's potential to its maximum and clearing the path for a more vibrant, healthy future.

Examining the factors that can lead to mitochondrial malfunction

Examining the Engine's Cracks: Causes of Mitochondrial Malfunction

Mitochondria are tiny power plants that are tucked away in the complex machinery of life, deep within our cells. The energy that powers our bodies is produced by these amazing organelles, which operate as fuel factories. However, problems may happen to any complicated system, and when these small engines splutter, the effects can be extensive. This is the tale of mitochondrial malfunction, an obscure cause of many long-term health problems, and a deeper examination of the variables that may lead these superpowers to falter.

The genetic code within us may carry traces of mitochondrial malfunction. Mutations in our own energy-producing coding, mitochondrial DNA (mtDNA), can interfere with these organelles' delicate functions. Conditions like Leber's hereditary optic neuropathy and Kearns-Sayre disease are severe examples of how genetic errors can impair cellular energy production. These mutations can be inherited or acquired over time.

The Triggers and Toxins:

Yet the story is not limited to DNA. Our surroundings have a significant impact on how healthy our mitochondria are. Misfunction can be brought on by exposure to pollutants such as pesticides, air pollution, and even some drugs. These elements frequently produce a deluge of harmful chemicals known as free radicals, which overwhelm the mitochondria's defense mechanisms and cause oxidative stress. The engines get weaker as a result of this stress, which reduces their capacity to generate energy.

Starting the Fire:

Even our lifestyle decisions have an impact on mitochondrial health, beyond chemicals. Chronic inflammation, which is a defining feature of diseases like diabetes and obesity, can interfere with mitochondrial function, setting up a vicious cycle in which decreased energy production feeds back into the inflammation. Furthermore, consuming too many calories, especially from processed meals and sugary drinks, can overwhelm the mitochondria, causing malfunction and making health issues worse.

The Chain Reaction:

Misfunction of the mitochondria can have far-reaching effects. Deficits in energy production can cause weariness, and trouble controlling blood sugar levels, which can further contribute to diabetes and obesity. Furthermore, the accumulation of free radicals can harm tissues and cells, causing inflammation and hastening the aging process. In severe situations, neurodegenerative illnesses like Parkinson's and Alzheimer's can even result from mitochondrial malfunction.

Exploring the Future Course:

The first step in lessening the effects of mitochondrial failure is to comprehend its causes. We may support our cellular powerhouses by making lifestyle modifications such as frequent exercise, a balanced diet, and stress management. Furthermore, research is also being conducted to treat the underlying reasons for dysfunction and maybe return these essential engines to full health. Potential paths of investigation include gene therapy, antioxidant medicines, and even mitochondrial replacement procedures.

Unlocking the full capacity of every cell means looking beyond the surface of sickness to examine the flaws in the engine. By illuminating the causes of mitochondrial dysfunction, we open the door to a day when these microscopic power plants can keep humming and support a more robust, healthy life for all of us.

Igniting the Powerhouse Revolution

Sparking the Powerhouse Revolution: Unleashing Our Mitochondria's Potential

Nestled amidst the complex machinery of life, the mitochondrion is a hidden powerhouse located deep within each cell. Often called the "engines of the cell," these microscopic organelles are in charge of producing the energy that powers each and every heartbeat, cognition, and bodily movement. However, as these titans falter and stall, a series of health problems may surface, leaving us to scrounge around in the dark for solutions.

The mitochondria revolution is about to begin, changing the way we think about health and illness. It's a tale of **releasing the tremendous potential that resides inside every cell** via the care and development of these essential engines. Mitochondria are assuming a central role in the pursuit of a more vibrant and health-conscious future.

<u>The Life's Spark</u>:

There's more to mitochondria than just energy production. They affect cellular signaling, metabolism, and even aging and apoptosis (programmed cell death). Because they have their own DNA, which is a holdover from their time as free-living bacteria during their evolution, they are vulnerable to damage and mutations.

<u>Using the Strength</u>:

The good news is that there is still hope for the tale of mitochondrial malfunction. We are deciphering the mysteries of these little powerhouses, opening the door to possible lifestyle changes and therapeutic interventions.

Lifestyle Optimization: Antioxidant-rich foods, regular exercise, and stress reduction all directly enhance mitochondrial health and function.

Nutritional Interventions: Certain nutrients, such as L-carnitine and coenzyme Q10, can improve the mitochondria's capacity to produce energy and protect against free radicals.

Emerging Therapies: To address mitochondrial dysfunction at its core, research is examining novel approaches like gene therapy, stem cell therapy, and targeted medicines.

<u>Exceeding the Person</u>:

The impact of the mitochondrial revolution goes well beyond personal well-being. Gaining insight into these titans of industry can lead to advancements in a variety of fields, including:

Aging and Longevity: According to research, enhancing mitochondrial activity may be essential for both encouraging healthy aging and prolonging life.

Diseases of the Neurodegeneration: Alzheimer's and Parkinson's disease are two neurodegenerative disorders linked to mitochondrial dysfunction. Novel therapeutic approaches might be made possible by acknowledging and resolving these problems.

Chronic disorders: Numerous chronic disorders are associated with mitochondrial dysfunction, ranging from autoimmune diseases and chronic fatigue syndrome to diabetes and obesity. New methods of treating these illnesses can be developed with the help of the knowledge gathered in this sector.

A Request for Action:

The goal of the mitochondria revolution is to empower people and societies to realize their greatest potential, rather than only curing illness. We may open the door to a future full of health, vigor, and a greater comprehension of the human condition by discovering the power hidden inside every cell.

Take part in the revolution. Set the internal powerhouses ablaze. Let us take one mitochondrial cell at a time and recreate the history of health.

Chapter 9: The Dawn of Mitochondrial Medicine

The Emergence of Mitochondrial Medicine: Revealing the Internal Powerhouses

They worked in secret for decades, their murmurs overpowered by the din of more recognizable machinery. But something is stirring in the quiet corners of our cells—a revolution. The cellular powerhouses, the once-overlooked mitochondria, are coming into their own and signaling the "dawn of mitochondrial medicine.

These microscopic titans are now acknowledged as complex maestros, controlling metabolism, signaling pathways, and even the very dance of life and death within our cells. They are no longer only energy factories. However, a host of chronic illnesses can develop, ranging from diabetes and neurodegeneration to autoimmune disorders and aging itself, when their delicate machinery malfunctions as a result of genetic errors, environmental pollutants, or the wear and tear of time.

<u>Changing the Framework:</u>

However, things are starting to change. Nowadays, mitochondrial medicine is a chorus resounding across labs and clinics across the globe, not just a whisper in the scientific background. Innovative studies are shedding light on these powerhouses' complex inner workings and opening the door for revolutionary therapeutic approaches.

Gene Therapy: Using the capabilities of genetic engineering, researchers are attempting to replace or repair damaged mitochondrial DNA, providing hope for genetic illnesses like Leber's hereditary optic neuropathy that were previously incurable.

Stem Cell Therapy: Patients suffering from neurodegenerative disorders like Parkinson's and Alzheimer's may be able to receive a lifeline from these cellular chameleons, as they show promise in rebuilding faulty mitochondria.

Techniques for Mitochondrial Transfer: * Researchers are investigating the bold idea of grafting healthy mitochondria into sick cells in an amazing display of cellular gymnastics, which could lead to a ground-breaking solution for widespread mitochondrial failure.

Medicine with Precision: Researchers are able to customize treatments for optimal effectiveness by identifying the precise genetic or environmental factors causing mitochondrial decline. This allows for the customization of each treatment to play a specific note in the intricate orchestra of cellular health.

<u>Inner Empowerment</u>:

The revolution is not limited to advanced laboratory settings. Common decisions can serve as powerful friends in the pursuit of ideal mitochondrial health.

Nutritional Powerhouses: We can directly promote energy generation and protect these small engines from the damaging effects of oxidative stress by loading our plates with foods high in antioxidants and mitochondrial cofactors like L-carnitine and CoQ10.

Fitness as Medicine: Frequent exercise stimulates the mitochondria naturally, boosting overall cellular health and acting as an engine. Stress Reduction: Persistent stress throws a kink in the delicate mitochondrial mechanism. Harmony can be restored, and its negative effects can be lessened, with the use of practices like mindfulness and meditation.

<u>Exceeding Personal Recovery</u>:

The effects of mitochondrial medicine go beyond personal health. It has the capacity to:

Fight Chronic Diseases: By comprehending and optimizing mitochondrial function, one may effectively combat a wide range of chronic ailments, from diabetes and obesity to neurodegenerative diseases and autoimmune disorders.

Extend Lifespan: Studies indicate that we may be able to live longer, healthier lives if we can achieve healthy aging and longevity through the maintenance of healthy mitochondria.

Empower People: People can reach their full potential and experience enhanced energy, vitality, and resilience by taking control of their mitochondrial health. This will leave them prepared to take on the day with renewed vigor.

The emergence of mitochondrial medicine represents a paradigm shift and a call to action rather than merely a scientific discovery. It's a call to action to pay attention to inner guidance, to cultivate the inner superpowers that propel our existence, and to rewrite the narrative of health one brightly lit mitochondria at a time.

Chapter 10: Gene Editing: Rewriting the Mitochondrial Code

Modifying the Mitochondrial Code via Gene Editing

Mitochondria are tiny power plants that are tucked away in the complex machinery of life, deep within our cells. These organelles are essential for metabolism, signaling pathways, and even aging; they are not merely energy producers. However, a series of persistent health issues may emerge if mutations in their distinct DNA take place. Herein lies the promise of gene editing, which holds the key to unlocking a future devoid of crippling illnesses by rewriting the mitochondrial code.

The Quiet Enemies: Mutations in Mitochondrial DNA

Mitochondrial DNA (mtDNA) is a circular, double-stranded molecule that is only inherited from the mother, in contrast to the DNA present in the nucleus of our cells. Toxins and oxidative stress are examples of environmental variables that can cause mutations in mtDNA that can be inherited or acquired over time. These mutations can cause serious disorders such as Kearns-Sayre syndrome, Leber's hereditary optic neuropathy, some types of diabetes, and Parkinson's disease by interfering with essential mitochondrial functions.

<u>Gene Editing's Promise</u>:

CRISPR-Cas9 and other gene editing technologies provide a breakthrough way to fix these mutations. Through accurate mtDNA targeting and modification, researchers may be able to:

Fix defective genes: The mutant mtDNA segment can be removed using CRISPR and replaced with a healthy copy.

Deactivate deleterious mutations: In certain circumstances, it might be more effective to "turn off" a mutant gene in order to stop any negative effects from occurring.

Explain more features: Even whole new genes might be inserted into mtDNA through gene editing, which might improve mitochondrial activity and general cellular health.

Difficulties and Points to Remember:

Although gene editing has great potential, there are still many obstacles to overcome. It is difficult to get the editing equipment to mitochondria, and it is essential to make sure that the precise targeting is done without causing any unwanted side effects. Regulations and careful deliberation are also required on the ethical issues of germline editing, which modifies genes that can be inherited by progeny.

A View Towards the Future:

The potential advantages of mitochondrial gene editing outweigh the difficulties. Leber's hereditary optic neuropathy is currently undergoing early clinical trials, and research into other disorders is ongoing. Gene editing has the potential to transform the treatment of mitochondrial disorders and provide hope for the millions of people and families affected by these crippling illnesses as technology advances and ethical issues are resolved.

<u>Exceeding Illness</u>:

Beyond curing current illnesses, mitochondrial gene editing holds great promise. Enhancing mitochondrial performance may allow us to:

Reduce the rate of aging: The long-term viability and health of cells depend on healthy mitochondria. Gene editing may help encourage healthy aging and slow down the aging process.

Improve mental clarity: Alzheimer's and Parkinson's disease are two neurodegenerative disorders that have been related to mitochondrial malfunction. Modifying mtDNA may offer defense against certain illnesses and even enhance mental performance.

Improve sports performance: For sports performance, energy production must be done efficiently. Gene editing has the ability to improve physical capacity and maximize mitochondrial function.

<u>Today is the Future</u>:

Gene editing is a fast-developing technology that has the ability to completely change the course of human health; it is no longer a sci-fi idea. Future generations can benefit from a healthier and more promising future if we can decipher the mysteries of the mitochondrial code.

Exploring the potential and ethical considerations of mitochondrial DNA manipulation.

Rewriting the Rules of Life: Investigating the Use of Mitochondrial DNA Manipulation in Ethics and Health

The microscopic power plants known as mitochondria are tucked away deep within our cells, amidst the complex machinery of life. These organelles are not merely energy producers; they also coordinate essential processes that affect metabolism, signaling pathways, and even the aging process. However, when their distinct DNA is tainted by mutations, a host of long-term illnesses may develop. Herein lies the power of mitochondrial DNA (mtDNA) manipulation, which not only has great potential to relieve suffering but also ignites important moral discussions.

The Influence and Danger of Deception:

 MtDNA modification includes a range of methods intended to rectify or alter mutations, which may provide treatment for diseases that were previously incurable. Among these methods are:

Gene editing: By carefully identifying and fixing defective genes, CRISPR-Cas9 and other instruments can restore mitochondrial function.

Mitochondrial replacement therapy (MRT): A potentially life-saving procedure for children with severe mtDNA abnormalities, MRT replaces damaged mitochondria with healthy ones from donor eggs.

Nuclear gene therapy: This treatment modality provides a less direct but potentially effective path by focusing on and modifying nuclear genes that affect mitochondrial function.

<u>The Hope Glimmer</u>:

It is indisputable that mtDNA modification has potential advantages. Gene editing-based Leber's hereditary optic neuropathy early clinical trials yield encouraging results, and MRT research gives critically ill children hope. Furthermore, modifying mtDNA might

Reduce the rate of aging: The lifetime and health of cells depend on healthy mitochondria. Enhancing the function of mtDNA may increase longevity and encourage healthy aging.

Improve mental clarity: Neurodegenerative disorders are associated with malfunctions in the mitochondria. It may be possible to prevent these illnesses and possibly enhance cognitive performance by manipulating mtDNA.

Improve sports performance: For physical performance, energy production must be done efficiently. Enhancing the function of mtDNA may improve physical capacity.

The Ethical Precarious Balance:

But great power also carries a great deal of responsibility. The ethical implications of modifying mtDNA must be disregarded.

Gene editing: Changing the mtDNA in sperm or egg cells may change the genetic composition of offspring, posing questions regarding unforeseen repercussions and the freedom to select one's genetic lineage.

Informed consent: To ensure that informed consent is genuinely achievable, patients thinking about these novel medicines must be properly informed about all potential risks and uncertainties.

Equity and access: There are worries that this innovative technology could initially be costly and difficult to obtain, aggravating already-existing healthcare disparities.

<u>Open Communication, Shared Experience</u>:

 Moving forward necessitates candid communication and cooperation between ethicists, scientists, decision-makers, and the general public. It is imperative that mtDNA manipulation be subject to strong ethical frameworks that give equal access, informed consent, and patient safety top priority.

In the end, investigating the possibilities of mtDNA alteration is a shared adventure that necessitates careful assessment of the ethical environment, not merely a scientific one. Through responsible navigation of this trip, we may unleash the enormous potential of these interventions, rewriting the rules of existence not only for individuals but also for the benefit of mankind as a whole.

Chapter 11: Mitochondrial Replacement Therapy: Replacing the Engines

Mitochondrial Replacement Treatment: Changing Gears for a Better Tomorrow

Mitochondria are tiny power plants that are tucked away in the complex machinery of life, deep within our cells. These organelles are not merely energy producers; they also control signaling pathways, affect metabolism, and even direct the intricate dance between life and death in our cells. However, a series of crippling illnesses may surface when their engines falter as a result of mutations in their distinct DNA. Herein lies the hope that mitochondrial replacement therapy (MRT) offers: a novel way to replace malfunctioning engines that may change the course of mitochondrial disorders.

Mitochondrial DNA (mtDNA), in contrast to the DNA present in our cell nucleus, is a distinct, circular molecule that is inherited only from the mother. MtDNA mutations can be inherited or acquired over time, interfering with essential mitochondrial functions. Numerous disorders, including Leber's hereditary optic neuropathy, Kearns-Sayre syndrome, several types of diabetes, and even neurodegenerative diseases, can result from these mutations.

Changing Gears, Bringing Hope Back:

MRT provides a novel method for treating certain mtDNA alterations. This is how it operates:

1. Healthy donor egg: To provide cytoplasm with healthy mitochondria, a healthy egg is utilized.

2. Nuclear transfer: The patient's DNA is transferred into the donor egg by removing the nucleus from the patient's egg.

3. Fertilization: Sperm fertilizes the resultant egg, which now has the patient's DNA and healthy mitochondria.

4. Embryo development: After being successfully transferred, the healthy embryo is left in the patient's uterus to continue developing normally.

MRT avoids the defective mtDNA by using healthy mitochondria from a donor egg, which may enable the embryo to develop normally and result in a kid free from the crippling symptoms of mitochondrial disease.

A Spark in the Distance:

Even though MRT is still in its infancy, it has great potential.

Treating serious mtDNA diseases: MRT may help youngsters with potentially fatal mtDNA mutations live longer and in better health.

Preventing transmission: MRT can prevent mtDNA mutations from being passed down to subsequent generations by utilizing donor mitochondria.

Creating opportunities for more study: The effectiveness of MRT may open the door for further cutting-edge mtDNA manipulation methods, hence increasing the range of available treatments for mitochondrial illnesses.

<u>Exploring the Ethical Terrain</u>:

But this ground-breaking technology also brings up significant moral questions:

Geneline modification: MRT alters the genetic composition of progeny, igniting discussions over its moral ramifications and the autonomy to select one's genetic lineage.

Informed consent: To ensure that informed consent is genuinely achievable, patients considering MRT must be properly informed about all potential risks and uncertainties.

Equity and access: Concerns regarding equitable access and the possible aggravation of healthcare disparities are raised by the high cost and intricate nature of MRT.

<u>A Joint Pathway to Better Tomorrows</u>:

Moving forward with MRT necessitates transparent communication and cooperation between ethicists, scientists, decision-makers, and the general public. It is imperative that strong ethical frameworks that prioritize patient safety, informed consent, and fair access direct its development and implementation.

MRT offers a ray of hope for families bearing the burden of mitochondrial illnesses, not only a medical advancement. We can use MRT to change the narrative surrounding mitochondrial disorders and provide opportunities for future generations by ethically navigating the field and guaranteeing fair access.

Understanding the promise and challenges of this emerging treatment.

The power plants of the cell, mitochondria, are crucial for both the synthesis of energy and the general health of the cell. But a number of variables can impair their function, resulting in mitochondrial dysfunction, which is becoming more widely acknowledged as a prevalent cause of chronic noncommunicable diseases (NCDs), including diabetes, heart disease, and neurodegenerative disorders. Maintaining their functionality and halting the onset of illness depend on mitochondrial communication and quality control. Our mitochondria's quantity and quality decrease with age, which can lead to a variety of health problems. Mitochondrial health can be impacted by stress, sedentary lifestyles, free radical damage, and exposure to pollutants, allergens, and infections. Thus, a promising approach to the diagnosis, treatment, and prevention of many diseases is the understanding and management of mitochondrial malfunction. Targeting mitochondrial changes is thought to be a critical first step in creating successful therapeutics, even if the precise processes and the causal link between mitochondrial dysfunction and NCDs are still being investigated. The potential of these essential organelles in preserving general health and well-being may be fully realized by investigating and resolving the issues related to mitochondrial health.

Chapter 12: Beyond the Lab: Empowering Your Mitochondria

Most eukaryotic cells have mitochondria, which are organelles in charge of generating ATP, the body's primary source of energy. The idea behind Beyond the Lab: Empowering Your Mitochondria is to enhance general health and wellness by promoting mitochondrial health. Numerous illnesses, such as cancer, neurological diseases, and cardiovascular ailments, can be brought on by mitochondrial malfunction. There are a number of strategies to maintain mitochondrial health, such as supplementation, a balanced diet, and physical activity. Boosting mitochondrial health has several advantages, such as enhanced immunity, more energy, and general health benefits. Case studies have demonstrated the potential benefits of mitochondrial treatments in the treatment of conditions like amyotrophic lateral sclerosis (ALS).

Discovering lifestyle interventions and dietary strategies to optimize mitochondrial health.

Dietary tactics and lifestyle changes are essential for maximizing mitochondrial health. Studies have demonstrated the ability of certain foods, exercise, and calorie restriction to support mitochondrial activity. Better mitochondrial health can also be achieved through dietary practices such as eating a balanced diet high in antioxidants, controlling stress, and upholding solid interpersonal bonds. Certain nutrients, such as CoQ10 and riboflavin, have been shown to help prevent oxidative damage to mitochondria and lessen fatigue. Exercise on a regular basis has also been shown to be an effective way to enhance mitochondrial function and general health. These dietary and lifestyle changes are crucial for promoting mitochondrial health, which can enhance general wellbeing and aid in the prevention and treatment of a number of illnesses, including cancer and neurodegenerative diseases.

For instance, physical activity has a crucial role in maintaining mitochondrial health without the use of pharmaceuticals by controlling mitochondrial quality control and stimulating mitochondrial biogenesis, according to a review paper published in Frontiers in Physiology. Furthermore, a study that was published in the same journal explores the connection between regular exercise and a healthy diet and how it may be able to slow down the onset of dementia and mitochondrial dysfunction in the elderly.

These results highlight the significance of dietary and lifestyle factors in preserving the best possible mitochondrial function.

To summarize, dietary strategies and lifestyle interventions, including exercise, calorie restriction, and consumption of a nutritious diet high in particular nutrients, are important for optimizing mitochondrial health. These strategies are critical for maintaining general health and could benefit the prevention and treatment of a number of illnesses linked to mitochondrial dysfunction.

PHASE 4

A Future Powered by Mitochondria

The idea behind "A Future Powered by Mitochondria" is that mitochondria have the ability to affect many facets of health and wellbeing. The energy-producing organelles of the cell, mitochondria, are crucial for ATP synthesis. The significance of mitochondria in aging, disease, and general health has been clarified by a recent study. One study, for example, showed that light energy could be converted by genetically modified mitochondria into chemical energy that cells might use. This finding could provide new information about mitochondrial dysfunction and aging. The Mito Food Plan also highlights the role that mitochondria play in aging and the onset of chronic illnesses, emphasizing how important it is to maintain mitochondrial health through dietary practices and lifestyle modifications. Moreover, studies have demonstrated the critical role mitochondria play in mental health, sickness, and even space biology, indicating the broad significance of comprehending and utilizing mitochondrial power. These results highlight how mitochondria may influence healthcare and wellbeing in the future, which makes this a fascinating field for further research and investigation.

Chapter 13: The Age of Longevity: Can Mitochondria Hold the Key?

The powerhouses of the cell, mitochondria, have been connected to aging and age-related illnesses. Studies have indicated a correlation between mitochondrial failure and a reduction in cellular function, as well as a heightened susceptibility to age-related illnesses. Because of the critical role mitochondria play in energy production and cellular respiration, dysfunctional mitochondria have been linked to a number of age-related illnesses, including cancer, cardiovascular disease, and neurodegenerative disorders. According to the notion of oxidative stress in aging, mitochondria are important players in the aging process because they produce reactive oxygen species (ROS), which can cause harm and a decrease in biological function. On the other hand, new research has also shown that a slight decline in mitochondrial activity can increase longevity. Age-related diseases and aging-related aging processes may benefit from strategies that improve mitochondrial quality and function, such as exercise, calorie restriction, and eating a nutritious diet high in certain nutrients. Understanding and improving mitochondrial health may be crucial to treating age-related illnesses and extending life, even if the precise relationship between mitochondria and aging is complicated.

The significance of mitochondrial DNA (mtDNA) in aging and age-related disorders has also been brought to light by recent studies. In contrast to nuclear DNA, mtDNA is more vulnerable to environmental stressors and reactive oxygen species (ROS), which can result in mutations and deletions that compromise mitochondrial function. Numerous age-related illnesses, such as Parkinson's disease, Alzheimer's disease, and cancer, have been connected to these mtDNA abnormalities. Furthermore, research has demonstrated that mtDNA mutations increase with aging, impairing mitochondrial function and raising the risk of age-related illnesses.

In a number of animal models, the possibility that mitochondria may contribute to lifespan has also been investigated. For example, research has demonstrated that caloric restriction, a dietary strategy associated with enhanced mitochondrial activity, can increase longevity in a variety of species, such as monkeys and mice. Furthermore, studies have shown that enhancing mitochondrial activity through genetic interventions can extend longevity in animal models. According to these results, maintaining mitochondrial health may help increase longevity and encourage healthy aging.

In conclusion, the function of mitochondria in aging and age-related disorders may have an impact on longevity. Although the connection between aging and mitochondria is complicated, studies have shown that it is possible to enhance mitochondrial health through dietary choices and lifestyle modifications in order to encourage healthy aging and increase longevity. To fully comprehend the mechanisms behind the association between aging and mitochondria and to create efficient therapies for enhancing mitochondrial longevity and health, more research is required.

Exploring the potential of mitochondrial medicine in extending lifespan and promoting healthy aging.

A new area of study called "mitochondrial medicine" looks at how enhancing mitochondrial health may increase longevity and encourage good aging. Age-related disorders are more likely to strike an organism because mitochondrial activity decreases with age, resulting in a reduction in cellular performance. Numerous age-related illnesses, such as cancer, cardiovascular disease, and neurological disorders, have been linked to mitochondrial malfunction. Age-related diseases and aging-related aging processes may benefit from strategies that improve mitochondrial quality and function, such as exercise, calorie restriction, and eating a nutritious diet high in certain nutrients.

The potential of mitochondrial therapy in treating age-related disorders has also been brought to light by recent studies. For example, a study that was published in the journal Aging Cell showed that an antioxidant that targets mitochondria can enhance mitochondrial function and lower oxidative stress in older adults, which may provide a novel treatment strategy for age-related diseases. Furthermore, studies have demonstrated that the procedure known as "mitochondrial transplantation," which entails transferring functioning mitochondria to cells lacking them, might enhance cellular function and lower the risk of age-related illnesses. These results imply that mitochondrial medicine may be useful in the treatment of age-related illnesses and in the promotion of healthy aging.

In summary, research into the potential of mitochondrial therapy to promote healthy aging and extend lifespans is an interesting field. It may be possible to prevent age-related diseases and aging by promoting mitochondrial health through dietary and lifestyle changes. Furthermore, new findings in the fields of mitochondrial transplantation and targeted therapeutics may provide fresh perspectives on the management of age-related illnesses and the promotion of healthy aging. To fully comprehend the mechanisms behind the association between aging and mitochondria and to create efficient therapies for enhancing mitochondrial longevity and health, more research is required.

Chapter 14: A Legacy of Empowerment: Taking Control of Your Mitochondrial Health

In the realm of medicine, there is growing recognition of mitochondrial medicine's potential to increase lifespan and promote healthy aging. Often referred to as the "powerhouses of the cell," mitochondria are essential for the synthesis of energy and general health. Studies have indicated a connection between heart attacks and mood problems, as well as other health issues and mitochondrial dysfunction. In order to help both the general public and those with mitochondrial illnesses, there is a rising emphasis on incorporating mitochondrial health into routine treatment. This entails comprehending the role that mitochondrial health plays in many illnesses as well as how it affects physiology, food, and lifestyle.

Numerous methods have been found to raise mitochondrial health, which raises general wellbeing and longevity. Consuming good fats, such as those in fish and olive oil, is one of them. These fats are necessary for the mitochondria to produce energy efficiently. Furthermore, particular supplements have been created to improve mitochondrial health and lower oxidative stress, such as resveratrol. Additionally, it has been demonstrated that modifying one's lifestyle to include frequent exercise and high-intensity interval training improves mitochondrial function and encourages the creation of new mitochondria, which eventually supports cellular energy production and general health.

People can take charge of their overall health and possibly contribute to an extended healthy lifespan by adopting a proactive strategy to maintain mitochondrial health through everyday lifestyle choices and prospective medical interventions. This strategy has potential for those who want to actively maintain and improve their health as they age, as well as for those who already have health issues.

Providing practical tools and resources for personal optimization.

The state of one's mitochondria is a vital component of general health, and it can be optimized with useful tools and resources. Through knowledge of the essential tactics for increasing cellular energy and encouraging longevity, people can take charge of their mitochondrial health. A few of the crucial therapies entail providing dietary support for important substrates for regeneration, such as B vitamins, magnesium, and coenzyme Q10. Furthermore, dietary restrictions or intermittent fasting can affect mitochondrial activity, as can regular engagement in a variety of exercise disciplines to increase mitochondrial biogenesis.

The health of mitochondria can be directly impacted by alterations in lifestyle and practices that promote cellular energy. For example, PGC1-alpha, a substance that enhances energy output by activating mitochondrial biogenesis, has been reported to be highly induced by exercise. Moreover, for the best possible health and function of the mitochondria, an anti-inflammatory, high-nutrient diet is crucial. Consuming antioxidant-rich foods and vegetables, omega-3 fats, vitamin C, zinc, magnesium, CoQ10, carnitine, creatine, and B vitamins are some examples of foods and nutrients that can help reduce oxidative damage.

Apart from modifying one's lifestyle, certain supplements like alpha-lipoic acid and CoQ10 can aid in mitochondrial optimization. These supplements have demonstrated encouraging outcomes in reinstating mitochondrial function. People can maximize their mitochondria and get the wide-ranging benefits of vibrant vitality and wellness by embracing the power of lifestyle changes.

In conclusion, implementing important lifestyle practices, selecting carefully what to eat, and thinking about specific supplements to enhance mitochondrial function are all useful tools and resources for individual optimization of mitochondrial health. Through the integration of various approaches, individuals can unleash the potential that is inside their mitochondria and proactively work towards improving their general health and energy levels.

Chapter 15: The Future Unfolds: Unlocking the Unforeseen Potential of Mitochondria

With new discoveries and technological developments opening up previously unrealized possibilities, the field of mitochondrial health has a lot of promise for the future. Once restricted to the specialized field of cytology, mitochondria are now found more frequently in a variety of fields, such as clinical research, biomedicine, the pharmaceutical, and cosmetics industries. The biomedical sector is full of promise because of the critical role mitochondria play in cellular and metabolic processes. As a result, novel technologies and interventions are being investigated with the goal of optimizing mitochondrial function and maybe improving general health and longevity.

Recent research has demonstrated the connection between mitochondrial failure and a number of age-related illnesses, such as cancer, neurodegenerative diseases, and cardiovascular ailments. This has sparked the conjecture that therapies aimed at preserving or enhancing cellular and mitochondrial health may also offer means of delaying the onset of age-related illnesses and lessening their effects. Because of this, there is an increasing focus on incorporating mitochondrial health into routine treatment and comprehending how it affects physiology, diet, lifestyle, and other illnesses. By doing this, promoting mitochondrial health may benefit everyone, not just those with mitochondrial illnesses, and help bring about a paradigm shift in healthcare and wellbeing.

The study of mitochondrial health and how it might affect lifespan and general health is an intriguing and quickly developing topic. The future of healthcare and well-being could be shaped by the incorporation of mitochondrial health into routine medical care, the development of new technologies and interventions targeted at optimizing mitochondrial function, and the potential that these developments hold to unlock.

Discussing ongoing research and future directions in the field of mitochondrial medicine

Significant progress in the understanding and treatment of mitochondrial illnesses is being made possible by ongoing research in the field of mitochondrial medicine. A greater emphasis on genetics-first approaches has resulted from recent research that has emphasized the relevance of high-throughput sequencing technology in changing the diagnostic algorithm for mitochondrial diseases. This change could lead to a more timely and accurate diagnosis, which would ultimately allow patients with mitochondrial illnesses to receive more specialized and efficient care.

In addition, there is an increasing emphasis on incorporating the concept of mitochondrial health into routine medicine, with particular attention to how it affects physiology, diet, lifestyle, and other illnesses. This strategy may lead to the creation of methods that promote mitochondrial health and everyone's general well-being, which could be advantageous to both those with mitochondrial disorders and the broader public.

Apart from diagnostic and integrative methods, current therapeutic research is investigating several approaches to treat disorders related to mitochondria. These include investigating pharmacological, non-chemical, and targeted genome editing treatments, as well as promoting faulty oxidative phosphorylation (OXPHOS). Research is also being done on the creation of possible therapeutic solutions for disorders involving the mitochondria, such as gene therapy and the correction of abnormalities in the heteroplasmic mitochondrial DNA (mtDNA).

With ongoing research efforts and a developing understanding of mitochondrial biology and its consequences for human health, the field of mitochondrial medicine has a bright future ahead of it. The potential of mitochondrial medicine to improve patient outcomes and advance our understanding of human health and disease is being realized through the manipulation of mtDNA, the development of targeted treatments, and the integration of mitochondrial health into routine medicine.

Conclusion

Final Thought: Unleashing Inner Power.

In summary, the investigation into mitochondrial health has been a trip of discovery that has revealed the complex inner workings of these minuscule powerhouses that reside within our cells. The strength within us is found in the health of our mitochondria. This revelation became clear as we dug further into the fundamentals of mitochondrial biology, investigated the dynamic mechanisms of energy production, and negotiated the delicate balance of mitochondrial dynamics and homeostasis.

We also investigated nutrition, activity, and environmental factors, realizing how important these are in determining how healthy our mitochondria are. As knowledge about the effects of oxidative stress and the profound relationship between aging and mitochondrial health grew, so did the significance of supporting these cellular structures.

Cellular health is mostly determined by mitochondria, which are impacted by environmental exposures and lifestyle decisions. The need for focused therapies and targeted interventions to protect mitochondrial health became clear as we examined the complex interactions between illnesses and mitochondria.

A comprehensive viewpoint became apparent when the importance of mitochondria was acknowledged at every stage of life, from early development to the difficulties associated with aging. Maintaining mitochondrial health is a lifetime endeavor that needs to be taken care of at every turn.

We also looked into the future, where new research indicates very interesting possibilities. The field of mitochondrial health research is developing, which may lead to new approaches and uses for existing ideas that could completely change how we think about wellbeing.

The main takeaway from this investigation into mitochondrial health is that taking care of our cellular engines is the first step towards unleashing our inner potential. Our decisions matter, from the combination of a good diet and exercise to being aware of environmental factors. Beyond just a scientific theory, mitochondrial health is a profound realization that gives us the ability to take control of our health and realize our full potential—the power found in the complex dance of mitochondria that plays out the symphony of life.

References

Ames, B. N., & Shigenaga, M. K. (2005). Mitochondrial decay in aging and degenerative diseases. _Toxicological Sciences_, 88(1), 25-35.

Chan, D. C. (2020). Mitochondria: Powering the cell. Academic Press.

Taylor, R. W., & Turnbull, D. M. (2017). Mitochondrial diseases. Nature Reviews: Genetics, 18(9), 589-605.

Journal Articles:

Atamna, H., Razaq, R., Ashraf, S., Hussain, A., Chandra, D., & Alwarth, S. (2022). The therapeutic potential of dietary and lifestyle modifications in mitochondrial diseases. _Frontiers in Pharmacology_, 13, 809549.

Gorman, A., Chowdhury, Z., Sinclair, D. A., & Mattson, M. P. (2015). Mitochondria as a therapeutic target for age-related neurodegenerative diseases. Nature Reviews: Drug Discovery, 14(7), 523-540.

Picard, M., Ritchie, J., Li, Z., Pawlak, M., & Taylor, M. S. (2018). Mitochondrial functions in metabolism and aging. Cell Metabolism, 28(4), 709-734.

Wallace, D. C. (2015). Mitochondrial DNA variation and human evolution. The New England Journal of Medicine, 373(15), 1428-1434.

Websites:

National Institutes of Health - Mitochondrial Medicine Society:

[http://www.mitosoc.org/](http://www.mitoso
c.org/)

MitoAction:
[https://www.mitoaction.org/](https://www.m
itoaction.org/)

The Michael J. Fox Foundation for Parkinson's
Research:
[https://www.michaeljfox.org/](https://www.
michaeljfox.org/)

About The Author

Dr. Dave Wilson is a seasoned explorer in the uncharted territory of mitochondria, those enigmatic cellular powerhouses that hold the key to our health and well-being. With years of experience under his belt, he has become a veteran researcher, shedding light on the complex interplay between mitochondria and rare genetic anomalies.

Imagine him as a seasoned spelunker, navigating the intricate caverns of the human cell, his headlamp piercing the mysteries hidden within mitochondria. His dedication to unraveling the secrets of these miniature marvels has not only illuminated our understanding of rare genetic disorders but also paved the way for potential treatments that could improve countless lives.

A Passion for the Puzzling: Dr. Wilson's fascination with mitochondria began early in his career, captivated by their unique role in energy production and their intricate connection to various cellular processes. However, his focus soon shifted to the perplexing world of rare genetic anomalies, where mitochondrial dysfunction often plays a central role.

Unraveling the Enigma: With meticulous attention to detail and unwavering perseverance, Dr. Wilson has delved into the labyrinthine world of these genetic anomalies. He has meticulously analyzed countless cases, searching for patterns and connections that could explain the diverse and often debilitating symptoms experienced by patients.

A Beacon of Hope: Dr. Wilson's research isn't merely academic; it holds the potential to transform lives. His findings have not only improved our understanding of these rare conditions but have also laid the groundwork for the development of targeted therapies aimed at addressing the root cause – mitochondrial dysfunction.

Beyond the Lab: Dr. Wilson's impact extends far beyond the walls of his laboratory. He is a passionate advocate for patients and their families, providing them with hope and a deeper understanding of their conditions. He actively participates in outreach programs and collaborates with other researchers around the world, his dedication fueling the momentum of progress in this critical field.

A Tireless Pathfinder: Dr. Dave Wilson is more than just a researcher; he is a pathfinder, a relentless explorer carving a path through the dense undergrowth of the unknown. His unwavering dedication to understanding mitochondria and their connection to rare genetic anomalies offers a beacon of hope for countless individuals and paves the way for a brighter future for all.